Make Ahead Paleo

Gluten Free Make Ahead Recipes For Busy People On The Go

Lucy Fast

Just to say Thank You for Purchasing this Book I
want to give you a gift <u>100% absolutely</u> <u>FREE</u>

A Copy of My Upcoming Special Report

*"Paleo Pantry: The Beginner's Guide to What
Should and Should NOT be in Your Paleo
Kitchen"*

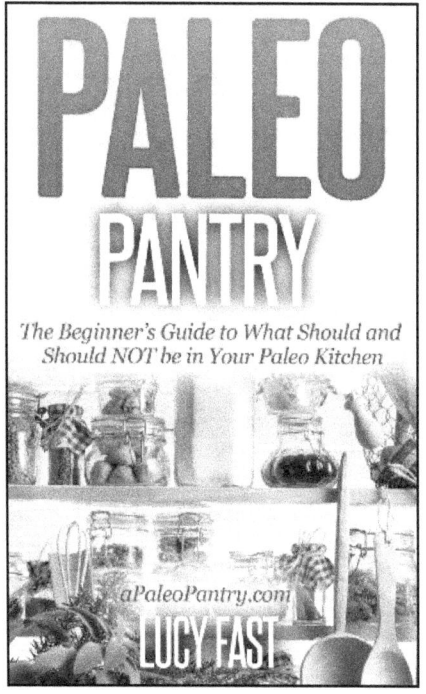

Go to <u>www.aPaleoPantry.com</u> to Reserve

Your FREE Copy

© 2014

Printed in the United Stated of America

Table of Contents

INTRODUCTION	6
TIPS FOR MAKE AHEAD MEALS	7
MAKE-AHEAD MIX: PANCAKES	9
QUICHE MUFFINS	11
TURKEY MEAT LOAVES	12
SPINACH-CILANTRO MEATBALLS	13
PALEO BURRITO SHELLS	14
PALEO MUSHROOM BURRITOS	15
WINTER VEGETABLE BAKE	17
HAWAIIAN BBQ CHICKEN	19
PALEO BALSAMIC CHICKEN	20
CHICKEN TACOS	24
PALEO RANCH MIX	27
PALEO MIXED-BERRY CREAMSICLES	28
PALEO CREPES	29
CHICKEN CHILI IN THE CROCK	30
HOMEMADE PIZZA SAUCE	34
FROZEN KERMITS	35
BRAZILIAN ICE CREAM	36
GELATO CHOCOLATO	37

CONCLUSION   38

CHECK OUT LUCY'S OTHER BOOKS!!   39

Introduction

In today's world, convenience foods provide quick meals for busy families on the go, but where's the nutrition in the drive-thru? It's certainly not over there with the added sodium in that meal-in-a-box or canned soup. Even most gluten-free, make-ahead options are packed with some kind of preservative or another.

Enter the world of Paleo Make-Ahead meals!

By making your own breakfasts, lunches, dinners, and desserts ahead of time, you not only save yourself time, but you also save money, not to mention the sheer amount of calories, fats, and preservatives you'll shave off your diet. Making your homemade convenience foods Paleo-style ensures that you're still feeding your family healthfully. You're aware of every ingredient going in that dish! In this book, you'll find ways to minimize your time in the kitchen that so you can maximize your time elsewhere. From sauces to mixes, sausages to popsicles, we've got your mealtime covered. Here are just a few of the dishes you're going to love:

- Paleo Burritos
- Gelato Chocolato
- Frozen Kermits
- Spinach-Cilantro Meatballs
- Turkey Meatloaf
- Cashew Chicken
- And more!

Let's move right along into the cooking, shall we?

Lucy Fast

Tips for Make Ahead Meals

Making meals ahead of time can be both convenient *and* fun. Here are some tried-and-true pointers for making the most of your make-ahead prep.

1. Make sure you have the right storage tools on hand.

Gallon-sized freezer bags and dishes that can go from freezer to oven are what you'll need for meal success.

2. Double up.

If you're making a casserole or soup, consider doubling the recipe so that you can eat one meal tonight and have one in the freezer for next week.

3. Make some mix-ins.

Along the same lines as the previous point: Why not grill a few extra chicken breasts or brown a bit of extra ground meat to store for future dishes?

4. Avoid the mush factor.

Avoid freezing anything that naturally carries a high-water content (think cucumbers, potatoes, and melons). Likewise, keep your Paleo Mayo in the fridge, not the freezer, since any egg-based sauce won't congeal when frozen.

5. Make some time.

It may seem counterintuitive, but a stitch in time really does save nine! Think about setting some time aside once a month to make a few meals for your freezer or mixes for your pantry.

6. Remember to label!

Whether it's pancake mix or ingredients for crock-pot day, note the creation date as well as any cooking instructions right on the bag or on a label attached to the storage container.

Make-Ahead Mix: Pancakes

Ingredients:

For the mix:

- 1 1/3 c. almond flour
- 1/3 c. coconut flour
- 3 T. coconut sugar
- 1/8 tsp. fine sea salt
- 1 tsp. cream of tartar
- 1 ½ tsp. baking soda

For the batter, add:

- 1¼ c. almond milk
- ¼ c. coconut oil
- 2 eggs, beaten

Directions:

1. Whisk together dry ingredients, and store in a large glass container until ready to use.
2. When ready to use, pour dry ingredients into a large bowl, whisking once again.
3. In a separate bowl, mix together all of the wet ingredients.
4. Add wet ingredients to dry, and stir until just combined

5. Heat a griddle over medium heat and spray with coconut oil.
6. Pour batter by ¼ cup spoonfuls into griddle. Flip when bubbles appear on pancake's surface. Cook for one additional minute.

Maks 10-12 pancakes

Quiche Muffins

Ingredients:

- Coconut oil
- 1 dozen eggs, beaten
- 1 lb. bacon, uncooked and chopped
- 3 cloves of garlic, minced
- ½ large red onion, chopped
- 1 large bell pepper, diced
- Sea salt and pepper to taste

Directions:

1. Preheat oven to 375°F, and spray a 12-cup muffin tin with coconut oil.
2. Fry bacon over medium heat until crisp. Discard all but 1 tablespoon of bacon grease.
3. Sauté garlic, onions, and pepper in pan until onions are soft and golden, about 5 minutes.
4. Add bacon and veggies to eggs. Whisk well.
5. Fill muffin tins 2/3 of the way.
6. Bake for 25-30 minutes.
7. Serve immediately or refrigerate for up to one week.

Makes 12 muffins

Turkey Meat Loaves

Ingredients:

- 1½ lbs. ground turkey
- 1 medium zucchini, shredded
- 1 medium carrot, shredded
- ½ Spanish onion, chopped finely
- ½ c. almond flour
- ½ c. salsa
- 1 egg, beaten
- 1 clove garlic, chopped
- Sea salt and pepper to taste

Directions:

1. Mix all ingredients together in a large bowl, kneading with your hands to make sure everything is incorporated well.
2. Form into one large loaf or three mini-loaves.
3. Place on a cookie sheet sprayed with coconut oil, cover with plastic wrap and foil, and freeze. Once frozen, wrap again in foil.
4. When ready to eat, thaw meat. Preheat oven to 350°F. Bake for 45-50 minutes or until done.

Makes 1 large loaf or three mini-loaves.

Spinach-Cilantro Meatballs

Ingredients:

- 2 lbs. ground chicken
- ½ onion, diced
- 1 tsp. sea salt
- ½ tsp. dried basil
- ½ tsp. garlic powder
- 1 tsp. cumin
- 2 c. baby spinach, chopped
- ½ c. fresh cilantro, chopped finely
- 2 eggs, beaten

Directions:

1. Line a baking sheet with parchment paper.
2. Using your hands, mix together, and knead ingredients in a large bowl.
3. Roll into palm-sized balls, and set on baking sheet.
4. Roll into small balls, and place onto prepared baking sheet.
5. Freeze meatballs in a single layer, then store in an airtight, freezer-safe container.
6. To cook, let thaw and bake for 25 minutes at 400°F.

Paleo Burrito Shells

Ingredients:

- Coconut oil spray
- 6 eggs
- 6 egg whites
- 1½ c. water
- ½ c. ground flaxseed
- 1 tsp. fine sea salt

Directions:

1. Preheat a 10-inch nonstick pan over medium heat.
2. Spray pan with coconut oil.
3. Whisk together all ingredients.
4. Loosen edges of burrito shell from pan once it's golden brown on bottom. Flip and cook on the other side for one minute.
5. Repeat until you run out of batter.
6. To freeze: stack one by one in layers of wax paper, and store wrapped in foil or in an air-tight, freezer-safe container.

Makes 6 shells

Paleo Mushroom Burritos

Ingredients:

- 2 T. coconut oil
- 1 large yellow onion, diced
- 4 cloves garlic, crushed
- 1 jalapeño, seeded and finely minced
- 1 large red bell pepper, diced
- 1 medium zucchini, diced
- 1 large tomato, diced
- 4 c. sautéed mushrooms, chopped
- 1 T. ground cumin
- 1 tsp. hot smoked paprika
- 1 tsp. chili powder
- 1 tsp. sea salt
- 1 small bunch of cilantro, chopped
- 6 Paleo Burrito shells

Directions:

1. Heat oil in a large skillet over medium-high heat.
2. Sauté onions until soft and golden.
3. Add garlic and jalapeños, and cook for an additional 2 minutes.
4. Add zucchini and red pepper, and sauté for 10 minutes or until mixture is soft and browning.
5. Add tomato, and cook for 1-2 minutes to heat through.

6. Add mushrooms, cumin, smoked paprika, chili, and sea salt, mixing well.
7. Divide the burrito filling between the six tortillas and fold.
8. Wrap single burritos in foil, and place in a single layer in the freezer.

Makes 6 burritos (1 burrito = 1 serving)

Winter Vegetable Bake

Ingredients:

- 1½ heads cauliflower, chopped into bite-size pieces
- 1½ heads broccoli, chopped into bite-size pieces
- 3 large carrots, diced
- 2 cloves of garlic, sliced
- ½ c. extra-virgin olive oil
- 1 tsp. dried basil
- 1½ tsp. sea salt
- 1 tsp. freshly ground pepper
- 3 tablespoons grass-fed butter, melted

Directions:

1. In a large mixing bowl, mix together all ingredients except butter.
2. Pour mixture into a 9 x 13 inch, freezer-safe casserole dish.
3. Pour melted butter evenly across vegetables.
4. Cover, and freeze until ready to use.
5. When ready to eat, preheat oven to 375°F. Uncover casserole, and bake for 1 hour or until golden and bubbly

Makes 6 (1-cup) servings

Paleo Cashew Chicken

Ingredients:

- 3 lbs. boneless, skinless chicken (breasts or thigh), chopped
- 1 tsp. pepper
- ½ c. coconut aminos
- ½ c. apple cider vinegar
- ¼ c. tomato paste
- 1 tsp. ground ginger
- Coconut oil spray

Serve with:
½ c. cashews

Directions:

1. In a large mixing bowl, add all ingredients, and stir together to make sure everything is incorporated.
2. Place mixture in a freezer bag with the following label: "Thaw and place in slow cooker on LOW for 4-6 hours. Add cashews right before serving, stirring well."

Hawaiian BBQ Chicken

Ingredients:

- 4 chicken breasts
- 1 c. tomato sauce
- 2 T. tomato paste
- 1 c. water
- ½ c. apple cider vinegar
- 5 T. raw honey
- 2 T. black pepper
- 1 onion, diced
- 4 cloves garlic, minced
- 1 T. ground mustard
- 1 tsp. paprika
- 1 T. lemon juice
- 2 c. pineapple chunks

Directions:

1. Mix all ingredients together in a large bowl.
2. Pour mixture into a freezer bag, and label with these directions: "Thaw and cook in slow cooker for 4-6 hour on LOW."

Makes 4 (1 cup) servings.

Paleo Balsamic Chicken

Ingredients:

- 6 chicken breasts
- 1 28-ounce can diced tomatoes
- 4 cloves garlic, minced
- 1 c. balsamic vinegar
- 2 T. extra virgin olive oil
- 1 tsp. sea salt
- 1 tsp. pepper

Directions:

1. Place chicken breasts in a large freezer bag, set aside.
2. Mix remaining ingredients together in a large bowl.
3. Pour tomato mixture over chicken.
4. Seal and label directions: "Thaw and cook in slow cooker for 4-6 hours on LOW."

Makes 6 servings

Pollo alla d'Italiana

Ingredients:

- 4 chicken breasts
- 3 T. extra virgin olive oil
- 1 large green pepper, chopped
- 1 large red pepper, chopped
- 1 large yellow pepper, chopped
- 4 stalks celery, diced
- 4 carrots, peeled and diced
- 7 clove of garlic, minced
- 1 14-oz can of diced tomatoes

Directions:

1. Place chicken breasts in a large freezer bag, set aside.
2. Mix remaining ingredients together in a large bowl.
3. Pour tomato mixture over chicken.
4. Seal and label directions: "Thaw and cook in slow cooker for 6-8 hours on LOW."

Makes 4 servings

Slow Cooker Bangkok wings

Ingredients:

- 2½ lbs. chicken wings
- ½ c. salsa
- ¼ c. cashew butter
- 3 T. fresh lime juice
- 3 T. coconut aminos
- 3 T. water
- 1 3-inch piece fresh ginger, peeled and chopped fine
- ¼ c. coconut sugar
- 4 cloves garlic, minced

Directions:

1. Place chicken wings in a large freezer bag, set aside.
2. Mix remaining ingredients together in a large bowl.
3. Pour salsa mixture over chicken.
4. Seal and label directions: "Thaw and cook in slow cooker for 6-8 hours on LOW."

Makes 8 servings (1 serving = 1/3 lb. wings)

Slow Cooker Sausage alla Pizzaiola

Ingredients:

- 2 lb. Italian sausage
- 2 large green peppers, sliced
- 2 onions, sliced
- 4 c. diced tomatoes
- 2 T. tomato paste
- 1 T. onion powder
- 1 T. garlic powder
- 2 T. dried oregano

Directions:

1. Place sausage in a large freezer bag, set aside.
2. Mix remaining ingredients together in a large bowl.
3. Pour tomato mixture over sausage.
4. Seal and label directions: "Thaw and cook in slow cooker for 6-7 hours on LOW."

Makes 4 servings (1 serving = 2 sausages)

Chicken Tacos

Ingredients:

- 5 chicken breasts
- 1 T. chili powder
- ¼ tsp. garlic powder
- ¼ tsp. onion powder
- ¼ tsp. crushed red pepper flakes
- ¼ tsp. dried oregano
- ½ tsp. paprika
- 1½ tsp. cumin
- 1 tsp. sea salt
- 1 tsp. black pepper
- 2 T. coconut oil
- 2 T. apple cider vinegar
- ¼ c water
- ¾ c. diced tomatoes diced
- 1 Spanish onion, diced

Directions:

1. Place chicken breasts in a large freezer bag, set aside.
2. Mix remaining ingredients together in a large bowl.
3. Pour spice mixture over chicken.
4. Seal and label directions: "Thaw and cook in slow cooker for 4 hours on LOW."

5. Shred chicken inside of slow cooker, and cook for an additional hour.
6. Serve with Paleo Burrito Shells

Makes 5 servings

Brownie Mix

Ingredients:

- 1 c. coconut sugar
- ½ c. almond flour
- 1/3 c. unsweetened cocoa
- ¼ tsp. fine sea salt
- ¼ tsp. baking soda
- ¼ tsp. cream of tartar

Add-in:
>   2 eggs
>   ½ c. coconut oil
>   1 tsp. of vanilla

Directions:

1. Combine all dry ingredients in a large bowl, whisking together.
2. Store in an air-tight container until ready to use.
3. When ready to use, mix together wet ingredients. Add to dry ingredients. Do not over mix. Bake for 25 minutes at 350°F.

Makes 1 mix (1 mix = 1 pan of brownies)

Paleo Ranch Mix

Ingredients:

- 1 tsp. dried dill
- 1 tsp. garlic powder
- 1 tsp. onion powder
- 2 tsp. dried parsley
- ¼ tsp. dried thyme
- 1 tsp. black pepper
- 2 tsp. fine sea salt

Directions:

1. Combine all ingredients in a small bowl, whisking together.

Makes the equivalent of 1 packet of traditional ranch mix.

Paleo Mixed-berry Creamsicles

Ingredients:

- 1 can coconut milk
- ¼ c. raw honey
- 1½ c. mixed berries (fresh or frozen)
- 1 tsp. vanilla
- 4 popsicle sticks

Directions:

1. Place all ingredients in a blender.
2. Blend on high for 1 minute or until berries reach desired consistency.
3. Pour mixture into popsicle molds and insert sticks.
4. Freeze, and remove when ready to eat.

Makes 4 servings (1 popsicle = 1 serving)

Paleo Crepes

Ingredients:

- Coconut oil spray for pan
- 6 large eggs
- 1 c. unsweetened almond milk
- 3 T. coconut flour, sifted
- 2 tsp. coconut oil
- 1 tsp. arrowroot powder
- ¼ tsp. sea salt

Directions:

1. Preheat nonstick pan over medium heat. Spray with coconut oil.
2. Combine all ingredients in blender, and blend until smooth.
3. Pour into pan in ¼ cup increments, and flip when top of crepe begins to look matte instead of shiny.
4. Remove from pan, and let cool. Repeat until no batter remains.
5. To freeze, stack in single layers with wax paper, and store in foil, freezer bag, or other airtight, freezer-safe container.

Makes 10 crepes

Chicken Chili in the Crock

Ingredients:

- 1 lb. chicken breasts
- 2 14.5-oz. cans diced tomatoes
- 1½ c. mushrooms, diced
- 2 c. chicken broth
- 1 medium onion, chopped
- 3 medium carrots, chopped
- 3 garlic cloves, chopped
- 1 bay leaf
- 2 tablespoons parsley
- 1½ tsp. sea salt
- 1 tsp. pepper

Directions:

1. Place all ingredients in the slow cooker insert. Cook for 6-7hours on LOW.
2. Remove chicken from slow cooker and place on cutting board. Shred using two forks. Return chicken to slow cooker.
3. Cook for one more hour on LOW before serving.

Makes 4-5 servings.

Chicken and Cauliflower Bake

Ingredients:

- Coconut oil spray
- 6 T. coconut oil
- 6 c. finely diced cauliflower
- 2 cups sliced fresh mushrooms
- 2 tsp. minced garlic
- 1½ c. coconut milk
- 16 oz. vegan Daiya cheese (optional)
- 3 broccoli crowns
- 5 c. shredded chicken
- 1 tsp. salt
- 1 tsp. garlic powder

Directions:

1. Prepare three 8x8 inch oven- and freezer-safe baking pans with coconut oil spray. Set aside.
2. In a large stockpot, melt the coconut oil over medium heat.
3. Add cauliflower, mushrooms, garlic, coconut milk, and half of the cheese. Cook until mushrooms are soft or cheese (optional) is melted.
4. Add the rest of the ingredients, and cook an additional five minutes, stirring frequently.
5. Spread mixture evenly among the three pans. Add remaining cheese (if using). Freeze until ready to use.

6. When ready to bake, thaw completely, remove any lids, and preheat oven to 350°F. Bake until casserole is heated throughout and broccoli is tender, about 30 minutes.

Makes 3 8x8 inch casseroles.

Breakfast Sausage Patties

Ingredients:

- 5 thick slices of nitrate-free bacon, cooked and drained
- ¾ c. chopped leeks, white ends only
- 1 medium apple, peeled, cored, and quartered
- 1 T. fresh rosemary
- 2 T. fresh sage leaves, chopped
- 1 T. molasses
- 3 tsp. apple cider vinegar
- ½ tsp. black pepper
- 1½ tsp. sea salt
- ¼ tsp. ground cloves
- 1/8 tsp. ground red pepper (cayenne)
- 2 lbs. ground pork

Directions:

1. Place all ingredients (through cayenne) into food processor. Process for minutes or until ingredients are finely processed and chopped.
2. Add pork, and pulse until combined.
3. Form into patty shapes on a large baking sheet. Freeze for 2-3 hours, and store in a large freezer storage bag.
4. To eat, fry in a skillet sprayed with coconut oil, or bake at 350°F for half an hour.

Makes 16 patties

Homemade Pizza Sauce

Ingredients:

- 4 T. pure olive oil
- 2 green peppers, chopped
- 2 heads of garlic, peeled and minced
- 2 yellow onions, peeled and diced
- 20-25 tomatoes, chopped
- 1 bunch basil, shredded
- 4 smalls cans of tomato paste
- 2 T. dried oregano
- 2 T. coconut sugar
- Sea salt and black pepper to taste

Directions:

1. Heat olive oil in a large stockpot over medium-high heat.
2. Add chopped tomatoes. Stir and cook until simmering.
3. Add basil, tomato paste, oregano, sugar, salt, and pepper, and reduce heat to medium-low.
4. Cover pot, and simmer for two to three hours.
5. Let cool, and blend with an immersion blender.
6. Ladle into 1-quart freezer containers or bags.

Makes 5 quarts

Frozen Kermits

Ingredients:

- 2 c. frozen chopped spinach, thawed
- 1 c. carrot juice
- 2 T. fresh lemon juice
- 1 mango, chopped
- 2 overripe bananas, chopped
- ½ avocado, peeled and mashed

Directions:

1. Blend all ingredients on high speed for three minutes or until smooth.
2. Pour mixture into freezer popsicle molds, add sticks, and place in freezer for five hours or until solid.

Makes 4-6 popsicles

Brazilian Ice Cream

Ingredients:

- 2 overripe plantains
- ⅓ c. Coconut cream
- 1 T. vanilla
- 1 tsp. cinnamon
- 2 T. carob

Directions :

1. Blend all ingredients in a blender until completely smooth.
2. Pour into a metal baking dish, and freeze for 30 minutes.
3. Scrape mixture back into blender, blend again, and freeze until you reach the desired consistency.

Makes 2 cups of ice cream (1 serving = ½ cup)

Gelato Chocolato

Ingredients:

- 10 oz. dark chocolate
- 1 c. water
- 2½ cups water (1 cup hot or room temperature and 1 1/2 cups ice water)
- 6 egg yolks, beaten
- 2 tsp. pure vanilla extract
- 1/8 tsp. fine sea salt
- 1½ c. ice water

Directions:

1. Place chocolate and water in the top of a double boiler. Stir constantly until melted.
2. In a separate bowl, add ¼ c. of chocolate mixture to eggs. Stir, and add another ¼ cup. Stir again, and return all of egg mixture to the chocolate. Stir to combine.
3. Blend chocolate along with all remaining ingredients (except ice water) in a blender on low. Slowly pour in ice water until all is blended.
4. Churn in your ice cream maker, and freeze in a freezer-safe container for two hours.

Makes 6 cups.

Conclusion

As you can see, making from-scratch convenience foods isn't as inconvenient as it sounds! Also, you get to add in the idea that you're saving money, providing nutrition, and avoiding having to deal with the "healthiest option" at the fast food place (or more packaging from the grocery store). Best of all, you've gotten rid of that *"Oh no, I still have to make dinner!"* feeling that has always plagued you on busy days! You might just get even more hooked on home cooking the Paleo way.

Lucy Fast

Check out Lucy's other books!!

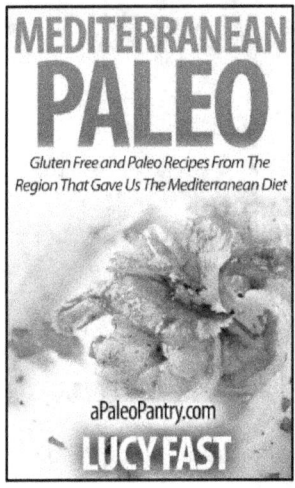

http://www.amazon.com/dp/B00JV4FNXU

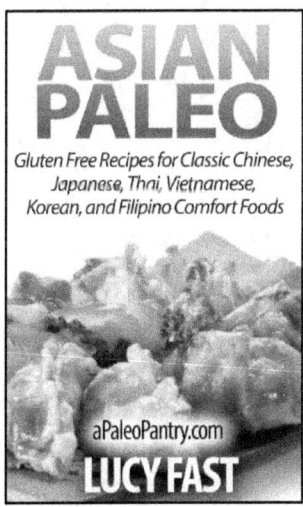

http://www.amazon.com/dp/B00JOS53H4

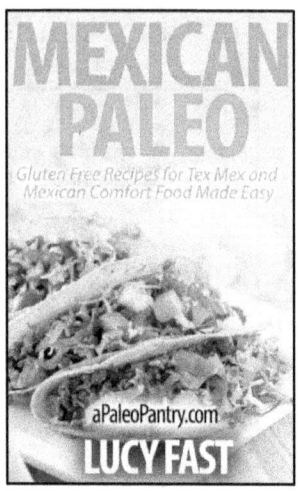

http://www.amazon.com/dp/B00J1UOLMI

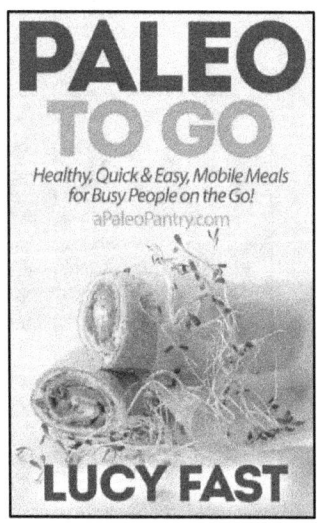

http://www.amazon.com/dp/B00HH1GBLC

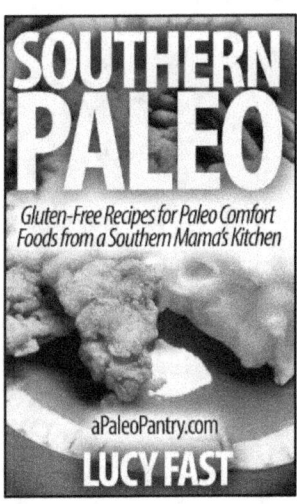

http://www.amazon.com/dp/B00HYKJCZ8

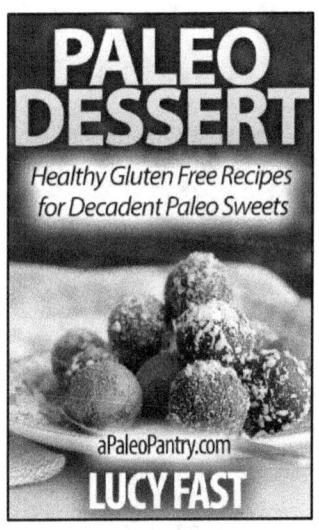

http://www.amazon.com/dp/B00JOWF758

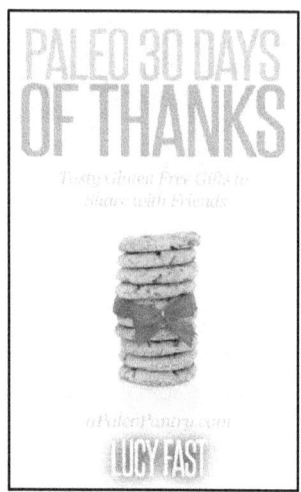

http://www.amazon.com/dp/B00OI0AUQW

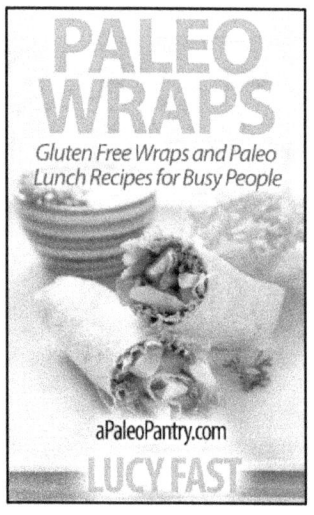

http://www.amazon.com/dp/B00IIHKA84

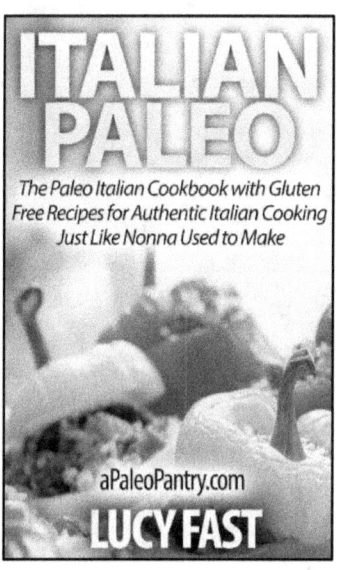

http://www.amazon.com/dp/B00J1TU18C